Dr. J. S. Roberts
I's
Guide to Weed

Published by
Nervana LC
Publishing

Dr J. S. Roberts I's

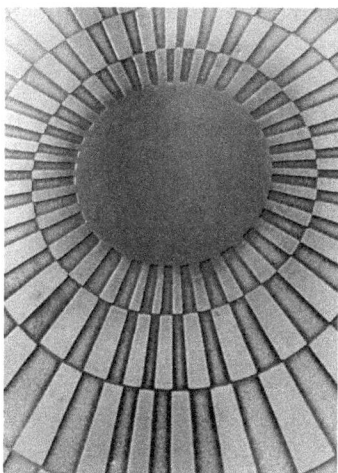

Guide to
Weed

Fall 2010

WEED

Cannabis Sativa/Indica

Description

Weed is a very old plant. There is evidence that people used it thousands of years ago. Today, humans are rediscovering its' usefulness and safety, and opinions about it are beginning to change.

It's about time.

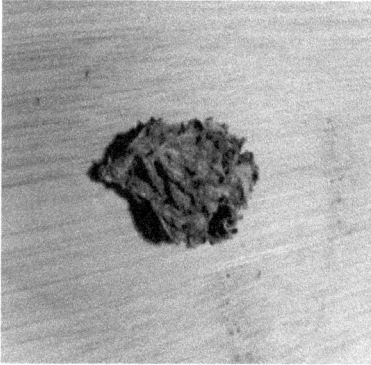

Bud

The main ingredient
in weed is a chemical
called THC.   This
chemical is produced
by the plants' flowers
in a sticky resin.

When the plant fully matures these flowers, or "buds", are picked, dried, de-leaved and prepared in a variety of ways for human use.

Some types of weed are grown without allowing pollination and do not produce seeds. This makes the buds bigger and they produce more THC.

Use

Weed has been used as a mind-enhancing drug for thousands of years. It also has been used as medicine and in religious practice for thousands of years.

It is safe enough to be grown and used at home.

There are many ways of using it based on personal preference.

Some of the more popular ways include smoking, bongs or water-pipes, vaporization, or simply eating it.

Smoking

To smoke weed a grinder or other device for cutting the weed into small pieces may be used and the result is usually hand rolled into a blunt, or joint. This is then lit and inhaled.

Although by far the cheapest, this is the least healthy option.

Bongs

Bongs are usually made out of glass, but can come in a variety of materials and a *wide* variety of shapes. These weed tools are made of a chamber at the bottom that is filled with clean water, with a tube like a round chimney attached.

There is usually a cup, or "bowl", with a tube at one end that slides down into the water chamber by a hole.

Weed is placed in the bowl and lit as the person inhales while pressing the upper end of the "chimney" to their mouth.

Proper timing of lighting and inhaling are key to this method. Bongs are also not a completely healthy option and they range from inexpensive to quite costly.

Vaporizers

A vaporizer is a weed heater that is attached to a fan. The fan blows air through the heater, the hot air is blown thru the weed, and finally into a bag or mouth attachment.

These devices can be a variety of shapes. They are healthier to use because they do not actually burn any weed, only heat it until the THC evaporates (or vaporizes).

When they were first introduced vaporizers were very expensive, however there are now many reasonably priced models.

Eating

Weed can be eaten. Many recipes exist for making all types of deserts, dishes, candies, etc. This is another cheap, yet healthy option for usage.

Effects

Weed alters the sensation of reality in favor of relaxed and easy going moods. It causes a slightly faster heartbeat. Mouth dryness, mild eye redness, relaxedness and laughing are often experienced.

There is mild short-term recall and memory loss while using that gradually reverses to normal once the weed wears off.

When used some experience anxious feelings or paranoia.

The way the weed is used controls how fast the effects are felt.

Smoking/bongs are the fastest at 5 to 10 min.

Vaporizers follow at 7 to 12 minutes.

Eating takes the longest at anywhere from 30 minutes to 1 and a half hours for effects to be felt.

The effects last anywhere from 3 to 7 hours depending on the weeds' strength.

Weed risks

The majority of risk with using weed is based on *how* it's used.

Smoking is harmful to lungs.

Use through vaporization has no great risks.

Eating has no risk.

Weed should not be used in the first trimester of pregnancy. It should never be used during activities that require attention, such as driving, operating heavy machinery, supervising children, etc.

It *is* safe enough for home use to personal preference.

Therapy

Weed has many benefits.

The most important is protecting the brain from damage.

It can relieve pain and muscle spasm(s).

Weed helps prevent dementia and damage from strokes.

It also reverses the growth of some cancers.

Weed decreases inflammation and is helpful in relieving headaches.

It can help with focusing attention and is extremely useful in disturbances of sleep.

Use is common for help with nausea, and many chronic pain disorders.

Author biography

Dr J. S. Roberts I is a board certified neurologist who has developed this guide after thorough history, scientific and clinical data, and comparison review with currently accepted federal guidelines for substance safety.

The words written here are his.

NERVANA LC
PUBLISHING

ISBN 978-0615996226

www.ingramcontent.com/pod-product-compliance
Lightning Source LLC
Chambersburg PA
CBHW021344290326
41933CB00037B/727